# WAKE ME UP

*A heartfelt story of one mother's battle
with postnatal depression and her
daughter's autism spectrum disorder*

## CLAIRE O'CONNELL GISSARA

This book was written entirely with one finger
in my notes section of my iphone. It was
written between midnight and dawn.

**WAKE ME UP**
**Claire O'Connell Gissara**

First published in Australia by Claire O'Connell Gissara 2019

A catalogue record for this book is available from the National Library of Australia

ISBN: 978-0-6484813-0-0 (pbk)
ISBN: 978-0-6484813-1-7 (ebk)

Typesetting and design by Publicious Book Publishing
Published in collaboration with Publicious Book Publishing
www.publicious.com.au

**Disclaimer**
This book is not intended as a substitute for the medical advice of your General Practitioner (GP). The information in this book is designed to provide helpful information on the subjects discussed. The reader should regularly consult a GP in matters relating to his/her child's health and particularly concerning any symptoms that may require diagnosis or medical attention. The publisher and author are not liable for any damages or negative consequences from any treatment, action, application or preparation to any person reading or following the information in this book.

*This book is dedicated to my family.*
*Bruno my one true and only love.*
*Max my only son who amazes me every day.*
*Mia my only daughter who amazes me too.*
*You are all my reason to live.*
*How blessed I truly am.*

# Introduction

I'm a simple woman. Some might say otherwise; in fact, I can guarantee that some might say I'm far from simple and they would even go so far as to say I'm borderline crazy! I make no claim of great intelligence as I share my story. I make no commitment not to swear here, but I do promise to write from my heart with the hope that other mothers feel a sense of hope in knowing that we are all doing our best during whatever challenges we face and that we can allow ourselves to admit when we feel broken and that it's okay to fall in a heap and ask for help.

I promise to share with you my story of fighting and of never giving up on finding an answer for my daughter's health and behavioural issues and her eventual diagnosis of autism spectrum disorder (ASD). I promise to tell you of the raw dreadful feelings I felt at 2am when holding my baby who had been screaming in inconsolable pain for hours on end and vomiting each feed until there was only bile left to bring up. When there was literally no sleep for her whilst dealing with this relentless pain and continual agitation of not feeling comfortable. I promise you that I will share everything as it will help us feel whole and connected in some way and in that comes great healing – knowing that universally we are one and love and time and friends and family can help you feel whole again.

I am simple in my romantic love of life. I'm simple in my love for my children and in striving to create a harmonious home. I'm a typical Cancerian: domestic, nurturing and kind, moody and emotional. I'm simple in my love of nature and in not being in any hurry to keep up with the socialites of the world, the latest trends or the hairstyle I should be sporting this month. I'm simply just a girl who grew into a teenager and rushed through my twenties without stopping to contemplate the impact of my decisions.

I became a mother to my firstborn son at twenty-seven years of age. I got divorced at twenty-eight and ran as fast as I could back to my first love who I married in my early thirties. Where does the time go? It's as if I'm still that young girl at twenty-two, handling my parents' divorce, still trying to find the perfect job and finish that three-year course. You wake up one day and it dawns on you that you're actually an adult dealing with adult issues.

Parenthood has to be one of the most incredible responsibilities one could dream of and one of the most rewarding and challenging. Suddenly your time is not your own – unless you're on the toilet, and even then it's almost always going to be interrupted with a little voice saying: "Mummy change nappy too?" The time you once had doing whatever you wanted is suddenly stripped from you as you juggle work, partner, money, kids, housework, and the occasional shag – and watching TV becomes your newfound obsession. Yet it's all worth it as you're totally in awe of your children with their skin that is so kissable as you dry them with their soft bath towel and that feeling when they touch your face and kiss your cheek.

Life becomes busy, exciting, harder and more stressful as you try to get your body back, cook nice dinners, and wash your husband's jocks with skiddies in them (how come I didn't notice that at the beginning of our relationship?!). You're busy trying to continue your career as even that is fading away into the past. We are all married. We are all committed. Life is hard enough when you're raising young children but what if something happens that you're not prepared for? What if you can't fall pregnant? What if you miscarry? What if your health fails? What if you lose your job? What if someone you love is diagnosed with a condition or illness? Is it the stronger ones who just cope better and battle on, or those like myself who are more emotionally sensitive who fall in a heap and can't get up?

Well, I've met my fair share of tough cookies and let me tell you, there's a breaking point in all of us, a point where we literally break. Your heart breaks and it's awful. Whether you admit it or not life gets in the way and damages you. It cracks your spirit and all that you can really hope for is the compassion and love of those around you to help you through. Compassionate people who know what you're going through as they have struggled too and someone somewhere once picked them up and so the universal love thing we try to understand starts spinning, and you feel hope again that you can get through it. That or a bloody big dose of Zoloft in the morning. Then you fight for your life and for those lives you created.

THIS IS MY FIGHT. ME. I'm thirty-six and three quarters, married to the love of my life with a ten-year-old son Max and a two-and-a-half-year-old daughter Mia. Max is from my first marriage, which lasted eleven months and Mia is from my husband now, Bruno. I don't ever plan on divorcing again (much to the disappointment of my mothers' group girls who hang shit on me that I've had two hens nights and two weddings all under five years!). I want to grow old and happy with the man who stole my heart at sixteen. Finding my first love again after twelve years apart is just so wonderful as not many can say they fell in love twice with the same person. So here is my story of falling in a heap and breaking, my story of motherhood and my story of illness and getting back up and fighting.

# Chapter 1
## Womb Time

I felt it! Like tiny champagne bubbles in my tummy! The connection between my unborn child and me was like a song only we sang that no one else could hear. I saw in the eyes of other mothers that they too have felt these champagne bubbles and I could tell they knew that I had no idea yet about the love my partner and I were about to experience together.

Being pregnant was the bomb. I had ten new books to completely submerge in from the beginning until week forty! I had hours and hours of time to learn about what was going on in my body at every stage! What the hell did I do with all my time before? The daydreaming was almost certainly interrupting my daily life; for the life of me I couldn't stop obsessing over my baby: what will you look like? What will I name you? My waist was expanding, and so was my heart. Nine months were going on like nine years as I waited to meet my baby. Life was going to be perfect in every way from that moment on.

Oh shit. The vomiting and nausea, the swelling, the sleepless nights, the muscles in my stomach stretching and feeling like they were being sliced with a knife as I turned in bed were all exhausting, but I was so happy and I kept going. This must be the beginning of sacrifice, I thought, the sacrifice for this unborn child as I will do anything and endure whatever it takes from the moment I get to take my baby bag to delivery and finally dress my baby in all the clothes I've bought for him (I knew it was a boy. I felt it and saw him in my dreams. Believe me, we know this stuff, us mums).

My journey to motherhood began and I joyously watched my husband also dream of this life-changing event of meeting our child.

Labour – got that down pat. No drugs, no caesar. I'm tough and I can do this on my own. I'll float through it all, said my naive self. I'll pop you out naturally, place you lovingly on my breast and you will feed perfectly just like my best friend Sharee's experience with her little son. Sharee made it look like a walk in the park even as I realised deep down that we all have different babies in our arms. I assumed I was equipped to handle anything. I had my superwoman cape on and every bloody item from Baby Bunting I could possibly need. I even had nappy bags that clipped onto the pram next to the doggie poop bags from the supermarket, such unnecessary amounts of wasted plastic.

Well, labour finally arrived and Jesus Christ why didn't any of you mothers with the champagne bubbles in your eyes let me in on the HELL of labour?! Never was I prepared for the pain to be so bad that attempting to suck on the gas was just too impossible in between horrendous contractions that momentarily made me believe I would die. Why didn't my mother say to me: "Breastfeeding is so hard you're better off with a bottle, love?" Didn't anyone think to tell me my vagina might be stitched up and my arse would need a medical icy pole on it for the swelling?!

So there I was back in the ward, icy pole in my pants with a maternity pad the size of a queen-sized mattress in my granny undies. But hey, I was holding our son. Our son who we named Max as we both loved this name before he was conceived and which means 'greatest'. My perfectly created son all of seven pounds two ounces, and life as I know it changed forever.

I stumbled through the next two weeks with highs and lows. I couldn't feed him and my nipples were bleeding, and I cried tears for my last attempt at it and gave up. Formula it was, and my baby was full, sleeping better than ever and finally pooping well. I learnt my first lesson that none of this parenting stuff is easy and I can't control it all, but hey I was still so proud and in love. I couldn't wait to dress him up and show him off at the shops. I was so happy going up the escalator I could've burst! I don't think anyone saw my ridiculous effort to open the pram in the car park – shit it looked so easy at Baby Bunting! I almost floated around like an angel on a cloud at the shops, enjoying my pram, my nappy bag and my newfound role as a mother.

Max was a textbook baby, and I put it all down to my experience as a childcare assistant and nanny having worked in Toorak, one of Melbourne's richest suburbs. I was organised and punctual and had everything in order. My perfect baby was never sick, which must be because of my wonderful efforts, I thought. My baby slept twelve hours a night and never woke, which I thought must be all that nanny experience with multiples and all that practise I've had. I felt like an expert and was so chuffed with myself.

At mothers' group meetings I gloated a little as Max is easygoing whereas others were struggling a little. I know now I was a little too sure of myself as Max was easygoing, happy, affectionate and hit every single milestone on time. He even grew into a perfect one-year-old. Ever the perfect baby, he took his first steps on his first birthday.

Life continued to be a breeze with motherhood, but my marriage ended when Max was a week off turning two. Guilty was too nice a word for the feelings I had about letting him down. I'd ruined the little fella's future. He'd never done anything to disappoint me, and here I was moving into a tiny unit that carried so many stale energies in it with no air conditioning either. How would we go in our boiling hot Melbourne summers? I was to be a single mother. It was over. His daddy wasn't going to be there every night but he was going to help and I made a vow that I would nurture my friendship with his father, respect him and never let my feelings interfere with our son's life. This ended up not being completely possible as at times it was a choppy legal fight, but we came through and we moved forward.

Little Max continued to light my days. Potty trained at twenty-three months and in Bob the Builder jocks at night, he never wet the bed. He was happy, I was happy. We were from a broken home but not living in one. I studied beauty therapy to fulfil my dream and provide for our future. Lesson number two: wow I fell down hard but somehow Max kept me up, and we almost skipped together into this new phase.

Increbibly and by the twist of fate I found my first love again Bruno after twelve years apart and life was like a true love story. I was bubbly, I was healthy, I was bright and engaging. I meditated every night and felt great comfort in my connection to the spirit world. I began to connect with a part of myself I knew had been open since I was a little girl and I enjoyed my space and my freedom. Max went down at 6.30pm every night, and I was free to recharge my batteries, get lots of sleep and spend time with Bruno.

# Chapter 2
## Mothers' Group

It's all very nice having girlfriends in our lives. The ones we grow up with, the ones we meet out clubbing or at university. But when you become a mother you get to have mothers' group friends. If you're as lucky and as blessed as me they become your sisters and if you happen to fall and feel broken, you will be forever grateful for the universe handing you your child and at the same time through fate it hands you friends to journey with for life, like family. You also find school mums! Deliciously loving school mums and kinder mums who you can spend time with talking about your children.

Mothers' group is funny. There was a burnt out tired health nurse sitting in front of me with hair that's so frizzy she reminded me of a crusty old clown! She was wearing a very sensible skirt and blouse and tried ever so hard to make us feel like she was hearing our dribble for the first time. She helped and advised us if we were struggling and offered support. The most exciting part was when eight other sleep-deprived young mums stumbled in with their babies dressed in the latest Pumpkin Patch outfits with matching slippers, headbands and mitts. I could see that they were just as frazzled as me and we all began to unravel who we are.

Some hit it off straight away with their common careers and others looked like they might never have sex again. Then there was me: twenty kilos heavier, short hair and still wearing my Millers size

5

eighteen white top. I was horrified. I'm not supposed to wear Millers until I'm in my sixties! Sitting there waiting to connect with someone I chatted away respectfully, soaking up lots of advice but secretly I thought I knew it all as I was a professional childcare worker and I had it all sorted with my perfect Max. I think I was even the only one with makeup on!

Looking back now I had no idea how life can turn on a dime or that the challenges I would face over the next ten years would see me forever different. Not lost completely but forever different.

Girlfriends are precious and so important in a woman's life, we seem to be able to share our feelings in a way that is free and non-judgmental. I may be generalising a lot as I know we're not all perfect – hence bitching and drama! But we do tend to offer each other a deep comfort and affection that our sister souls need from time to time. If it weren't for my girlfriends I think I would have driven into a tree one dark night at 2.30am; I think I would have never forgiven myself for being a drunken embarrassment at a particular party; I think I never would have learnt about compassion and forgiveness had it not been for the love of my girlfriends. Knowing that you can also return that support can give your heart such joy.

I was in cruise control as a single mum with no money but a heart full of love and a passion for life so large I was at times overwhelmed. Becoming a beauty therapist was so exciting and I was living in a world of glamour, lipstick, waxing and manicures! I couldn't have been happier. I truly loved life and began to dream of my future with Bruno and how I would have two more children, get married and sail off into the sunset. Yet God and my angels had other plans. They had set me up for a fully charged emotional rollercoaster I wasn't strapped in for or ready for what was about to happen in my life and my family's.

# Chapter 3

## Bruno

When I was eleven I moved to Australia with my mother Sarah, my father John and my older brother Nathan. We emigrated from London to live a better life and be with my aunties on my mother's side. I was born in 1977 when my parents were nineteen and twenty-one and my brother Nathan had been born thirteen months earlier. In London we lived in a tiny block of flats in the East End and life was tough. So this rather courageous move to Australia was admirable of my parents at only thirty and thirty-two years of age and having never been to Australia before.

Time went on and I adapted to school in Australia. My parents grew apart increasingly due to my mother spreading her wings and my father's love of the pub.

I was sixteen and at a party one night and feeling shy when a young boy called Bruno had noticed me. It was the next day at our local cricket club when he came over and spoke to me. We met through mutual friends and his face was so familiar to my soul. It was so intense and romantic and each date became more special as he would go to great lengths to impress me. Each month on the thirteenth we would celebrate our love. My heart was instantly his. It embedded itself into the deepest part of his being, and I knew my life would never be the same. We were a mirror reflection of each other and shared the next two and a half years inseparable. Two feisty people fighting just as passionately as we loved. We drove each other insane with our passion and they were the most romantic days of my life. If I shut my eyes now I can still smell him and feel myself there in those moments of pure bliss. Young love, true love and real fire yet neither of us had the maturity to uphold our relationship.

At seventeen my parents separated and ultimately divorced, which made me feel like the life had been ripped from me. I lost all belief in true love. I lost the young girl in me, the one who believed in fairytales. I lost my foundation. I lost my family, And in turn, I lost my Bruno. I left him shattered and broken and pleading for me to see sense as I told him that one day we would get back together but that I needed a break. I wrote him a devastatingly long letter, which he still has today, explaining that I truly believed our love was meant to be.

I hurt this young man so badly that his heart would never quite recover and he would hold onto that hope and knowing that one day I would return. I spoke of him over the years, I smiled every year on his birthday and I missed his face.

I went overseas to work and met another man. That relationship ended and so I returned to Australia where I heard that Bruno had moved on and was engaged to another woman. On my return I drove up the road where Bruno still lived and cried for the love we had. I kept his picture in my purse for years and years but little did I know Bruno dreamed of his Clairebear. His Clairest of bears as he would call me. Our lives ran parallel and we would hear through the grapevine what we were both up to, but it was bittersweet.

One August day I was six weeks pregnant with my first child and not yet married or engaged. I was driving down our town's country road with the radio on and I reached the T-intersection where I wanted to turn right. I was first in line. On the other side of the road was a black ute with a trailer also indicating to turn right into the street I was on. The cars were busy flying past and neither of us could turn. There was my Bruno! Sitting in his ute. Our eyes locked and as he turned slowly he smiled and waved and I captured that moment as if in slow motion. My heart jumped out of my chest and I was left wanting more. Then as I pulled away I held my tummy and wished this was our child I was carrying. I pulled over as the adrenalin was burning through my skin. I felt my heart plummet to the concrete gravel and sadness consumed me. I had to get to work but later I was to find out from him that he drove home that day and paced the house looking out the window hoping I would do a U-turn and go to his house. He waited and waited but I never came. I cried and cried for two weeks forcing the pain to the back of my bleeding heart by telling myself it couldn't be. But a spark had ignited in us both and it would take the breakdown of my marriage and two more chance meetings on the roads to make me realise how much I still loved him and wanted nothing more than to be his again. Forever.

# Chapter 4
## Marriage

Our wedding was magical and we were living a fairytale. We bought our first home together when Max was four, Bruno got his Builders Licence and I became a bubbly beautician working from home and at the odd salon. We were ready to start a family and try for a baby. I had always known deep down I would have children with Bruno, I just didn't think it would ever be so hard to fall pregnant even after only six months of trying.

Max began his first year at primary school and I was at home just waiting to fall pregnant, but the year went on and still nothing. I had peed on thousands of tests and made jokes to ease the pain. I relied heavily on my very strong belief that spiritually a soul chooses its time on earth and that it will happen when the time is right, which was not for me to decide. I had Reiki counselling, Reiki healing, I saw a chiropractor who insisted the nerves in my spine were connected because if the spine is in line then the nerves connected to the ovaries would function better, and I visited mediums and hoped for that reading where I would hear a baby was coming.

Another full year went by and I was swimming in sperm, literally. I couldn't do more, physically, to help, and by now the stress was affecting me and taking its toll. I didn't lose complete hope as friends were urging me to seek fertility treatment, which we did. After being poked and prodded by a big white prong that reminded me of a vibrator, there wasn't much going on in my ovaries, so we monitored when my right ovary was about to release an egg and rushed home to make love! How strange it all felt as my soul kept saying this is causing more stress, baby will come on its own.

I was prescribed Clomid and this remains my first memory of going a little 'crazy'. I visibly remember screaming at Max for the first time over his messy room. I was enraged and shocked at the intensity of my anger. Looking back now I'm ashamed to say what happened next but I promised honesty! (How else are you going to know that the world we so often keep hidden about how parenting can push us to the edge is part of the depression creeping in or the fertility drugs we take that are impacting our core selves?) I flew out of my son's room and with my right arm I whacked the stereo clean off the cabinet in our family room. Smashed it to pieces. I thought, maybe I'm a nutter, maybe I'm insane. The guilt I felt had taken a bite out of my spirit and I rationalised my behaviour by reasoning that the medicine was driving me insane hormonally and because my friend had warned me about going 'psycho' on Clomid, so that's what it was.

Needless to say, I stopped taking it after three cycles and this I believe was the beginning of my hormonal imbalance. I wasn't interested in trying fertility treatment and sadly Bruno believed that maybe I had had Max as a gift to him as he might not be able to give me a child of our own. Yet I dreamt of a girl and felt she was very close but there was still no positive test result.

I visited Maria, my beautiful Reiki healer. She had become my angel and by just walking into her aura my whole being relaxed and her genuine heart would wrap itself around me and I became open enough to say so much to her that I needed to. I was a little concerned that perhaps subconsciously I had feared this pregnancy would create another marriage breakdown as the guilt of leaving my first husband was unbearable in regards to our son. I thought perhaps I had created a block around myself, as fear will do that!

So Maria and I talked and talked and shared a deep meditation to release any fear. Then as I lay on her beautiful butterfly massage table and shut my eyes and dropped my shoulders, I began to relax.

I could smell bergamot and lemon and my ears were gently comforted by the sounds of waves and flutes from her beautiful music. Maria didn't speak. She just held my shoulders lovingly for minutes – touch is a powerful thing and I was transported instantly to being a child and how I felt being comforted by my mother. I relaxed more and she told me there was a female energy around me. She could feel it as she made her way to my torso and just gently placed one hand on my stomach.

I felt and saw in my mind's eye a navy blue energy pulling from my left arm and then there was energy and a buzzing feeling in certain parts of my limbs. Maria finished by simply holding my feet. It was so lovely and I felt like a child again. I know we can't remember being babies but every baby feels the love in a sensory way so that must be what stays in our subconscious.

I sat up, sipped some water and actually cried a little for the feeling of relief in my heart. I told Maria that while I lay there I asked for my baby. I asked for her with an open heart and I saw her on a rocky waterfall in my mind. I swam up the river and my grandfather (who is still alive, by the way) was holding her. He had big wings and I took her from him. She was chubby and had thick black hair and big cheeks. I was skin to skin with her and my meditation was either a simple daydream or something more universally apparent. I chose to believe it was a sign. A beautiful sign to let go of the fear, dash my baby a spirit invite and be completely open to have her arrive when she wanted. I left feeling literally on top of the world. That same day I walked the lake and looked up to the sky and said I'm here and I'm ready. Little did I know I was four weeks pregnant already – go figure!

# Chapter 5

## Turning Points

It had been a long three years trying for our baby. The day had come and I can still remember it like it was yesterday. I remember who I was and how I felt that day. I just didn't know that day would be a day I missed and longed for three years on. My ride was about to begin. No seatbelt, just me in my blissful state of happiness at the arrival of life inside me again.

I stood by our dining room table in shock that finally that double pink line had appeared on the pregnancy test. I was wearing black cargo pants and a black zip up jacket, my hair was wavy and styled and I felt beautiful and comfortable in my skin. My faith in my spirituality had been restored as I never gave up hope that my girl would come. I rang Bruno without thinking and he was just as shocked. Being a first-time father he needed more proof and wanted a doctor to confirm it. But a test is a test and a double stripe means baby baby baby. I explained that HCG is a hormone only found when a woman is pregnant and that is what was detected. He just sounded like he had won the lottery but was scared it might not be true.

Our 360-degree turn was about to spin us so out of control. I'm still shocked that we're still together today. Bruno has seen me raw, open, bleeding, sick and depleted and at times very angry, yet he still loves me. I have seen him worry, fight and say the four-letter word (you know the one that starts with C not F) as he was frustrated, hurt, angry and lost. Yet I still see him as my hero and I only hope I'm still his Clairest.

# Chapter 6
## Pregnancy

Two weeks had passed and I was six weeks pregnant. I felt great and our family were overjoyed and our friends too! I woke up on a Tuesday and was exactly six weeks to the day when I vomited. I rang Bruno and he said, "Don't think about it and try not to focus too much." I was instantly worried I would be like I was with Max. I was ill and vomited about six times that day.

The next day every smell and every food made me dry retch and I continued to vomit from 7am until midnight. It was exhausting and I hoped and prayed I would hit twelve weeks soon and it would stop or at least settle down. I vomited day and night for a week until there was just bile and saliva left. I sipped ginger beer and ate three to six peanuts a day. I vomited and vomited continually so the doctors gave me Ondansetron wafers and Maxolon to help, which are both antiemetics.

Ondansetron is used for cancer patients after chemotherapy. It didn't really help me and I was so weak and pale and tired. I had blown all the blood vessels around my eyes and I took myself to the ER at twelve weeks where I was given fluids through an IV drip, which made me feel better.

My obstetrician said I had hyperemesis gravidarum, meaning severe vomiting in pregnancy. I remember googling the word hyperemesis and discovering that it's considered a rare complication in pregnancy, but because nausea and vomiting often exist in pregnancy it can be difficult to distinguish this condition from the more common form of morning sickness.

I remember a school mum saying: "Oh you just have to suck it up, we've all vomited." I walked home crying thinking this condition bears no sympathy and it should be called 'evil sickness'.

My body felt like it was rejecting every atom of our child. Every week I went to hospital to be given fluid. I arrived at the ER one night and was instantly seen to and given my first dose of Ondansetron through a syringe. For fifteen blissful minutes my body was relieved of its emptiness and sickness, the busy nurse who had forced the IV in half an hour prior with such force to get a vein, had come back with a meal on a light blue plastic dish with a lid. A fork and a knife in hand I lifted the lid. There was an excuse for gravy poured over dark thick slabs of unidentified roast meat, roast pumpkin bricks and potato too! As an added bonus it had mint sauce on the side (must've been lamb then!), oh and not to forget the best soggy peas in the world. Any other day if given this meal I don't think I would have been able to eat it, but never in my entire life have I enjoyed every delectable bite of a meal! I ate with fury and so fast I had to pause to giggle, smile and revel in my moment! I left nothing on the plate that night. I left with my script thinking that the wafers would do the same once home. They didn't. For $125 for four tablets they bloody well should have!

I continued to vomit every half an hour from dusk 'til dawn. When I reached four months my darling husband took me to Queensland to stay and see his parent's penthouse on the Gold Coast that they had recently purchased since retiring. Max came too and we arrived safely, but little did I know there was a problem with the rubbish shoots up at level 73 at the Q1 resort that we were staying at. I was not prepared for the smell leaving the lift and it still haunts me today. It smelt like a rubbish tip on a forty degree day. There was no escape as the wall to my ensuite was next to the bins. I spent the next ten days next to the toilet and next to the stench.

At sixteen weeks I was surviving on six or seven peanuts and ginger beer. We came home and I continued to visit the hospital for fluids. When I reached twenty-three weeks I had lost 7kg and I was worried how on earth our child was surviving, but my symptoms decreased and finally I ate a dim sim and a slice of cheesecake. I continued to vomit but only now and then. I was very big like I had swallowed a basketball. I was growing more and more each week and at twenty-eight weeks I looked like I was due. My fundal height was 36cm when usually at forty weeks pregnant it's 40cm from the top to the bottom of your bump. Give or take a few.

Off I went to get extra ultrasounds as I now had polyhydramnios, which is a condition where you have too much fluid. My fundal height was 54cm at forty weeks and I could barely stand as I had become so large. I went from 65kg to 103kg in seventeen weeks. I was to be induced.

I kept thinking, what the fuck is going on here? Can't I just be like that newsreader on TV who works up until birth and turns up back at work with her washboard tummy and looking better than she ever did? Why can't I be like that? I didn't want to be ungrateful but I felt like my pregnancy was killing me. I actually hated being pregnant, it's awful to say, but again here comes the rawness of my story, as one night I just cried and cried wanting to escape the body I was in. I just couldn't hold on anymore. But our baby was big and healthy in my womb and so I battled on.

# Chapter 7
## Birth

I'm sure you have gathered by now I'm a drama queen, hypochondriac, unhealthy, moaning, pain in the bottom. I was sick of it too. Every day I was depositing how guilty I felt for not coping into my negative self-talk account. I was even getting a reputation for being a little on the fragile side.

Little did I know then how warrior-like I actually was. My depression was kicking in already and I was told I would be induced on Tuesday 20 May 2011 with a 7am arrival at the hospital. The night before my induction I discovered what a stretch and sweep is. It's a term used to describe a procedure performed to get labour started. The cervix is stretched with the hope that the mucus plug comes away. Basically, your obstetrician's hand is inserted so far up into your cervix and then forcibly turned 360 degrees. Well fuck me. "Are you fucking right, Mister?" Jesus Christ, he had no idea how that will ever feel and given I had no verbal warning it was coming I wanted to matrix kick the shit out of him and his bow tie! I sat up and wept.

I couldn't speak and my lip quivered. He said, "Did I hurt you?"

"Just get me home, Bruno, please." We headed home ready to see the doctor in the morning. My plug fell away and natural labour started at home for me.

The next day when we arrived at the hospital the doctor used his knitting needle to break my waters and in the process left a cut on the top of our baby's head: two tiny red scratches and the motherly instincts in me wept, if I'm honest.

Midwives were to keep me on Pitocin until the third stage of labour. No need, dickhead, I'm a woman and my body is made to do this shit yet you insisted on stretching and sweeping me the night before. It's a shame the doctor induced me with drugs, only to leave my husband and me two minutes later and never to return (not even after the birth). I was then to endure a two-and-a-half-hour labour with twenty-two minutes of it being second stage. My body was forced with such horrendous speed to expel our child that my poor husband describes it as watching me die in a car crash where he couldn't save me. Moan moan moan, yes I know I'm going on, but if you have ever been in labour you may also feel that it's refreshing to read this as no one ever writes about the details. We just get the bullshit version of it all in the twelfth edition of 'Baby and Me' magazine!

I was in agony. Complete agony, and my body begged for that last burning push to give birth. With my hands gripped around Bruno's t-shirt, she was born. She came towards me like a gift from heaven.

She had the longest fingers, nothing like my tiny hands and I saw my mother-in-law instantly coming towards me as my baby was my husband all over. A female Bruno with dark dark hair and chubby cheeks. But she wasn't breathing and Bruno didn't get to cut the cord as they whisked her away to clear her airways.

Once she was breathing well and back with us she continued to cry lots, holding her breath for seconds at a time. It was most distressing to see and it just didn't stop. My buddy Pitocin and I delivered the after birth and my episiotomy was stitched.

Mia Claire Monique Gissara was born eight pounds eleven ounces at 2.02pm, which was three and a half hours after induction. We dressed her as my father John arrived, and my mother Sarah and my grandmother June came, too. Still in the delivery room, mind you! Holy crap I needed a shower. Back in the ward Mia was screaming and screaming, unsettled and uneasy. My colostrum turned instantly into full breast milk and I was to learn later that the antiemetics I was given can also be prescribed to bring on a mother's milk. I had enough to open a milk bar! Mia fed well and it was fabulous but she was still crying. All the other babies born that day were asleep after their tiring entry into the world and my four-bedder was silent. It was 2.30am, twelve hours after her birth and Mia was still very unsettled and I could feel the bubbles popping in her tummy.

The nurse offered to take her for a few hours and told me to sleep. At 5am they brought her back to me and told me she'd done her first stool and that she had been full of wind. She was peaceful for the first time. They also told me that she was a talker as she hummed and hummed like a Tibetan monk! The nurse then went on to inform me that they were very sorry but she had had her birth identity tag on her ankle so tight it had indented her skin and left a bruise. When they removed it she calmed down and fell asleep. Oh my god, I felt sick to my stomach realising that's why our baby girl had been screaming. I wanted Bruno and felt guilty about the tag being on too tight. My heart was weeping and I felt like a useless mother inside. Unless you become a mother yourself you can't understand that feeling of wanting to take away your child's suffering and bear it yourself. The mark was dark purple and red in colour and I ran my finger over it softly and that was when I held her and truly realised she was a little girl. She was here, my beautiful girl.

# Chapter 8
## Feeding

Mia remained the image of her father. It was scary. She was coming home to begin her life as our first daughter and a little sister for Max to love and cherish. She was strong in her presence and her eyes were always wide open looking around intently. I thought to myself, is this what Max did? I couldn't remember. She was so alert and when my friend Natasha (who happens to have triplets, so is a baby expert in my eyes) met her she said, "Claire, she's beyond a week old and she's staring at me!"

Mia was having a lot of trouble keeping her feeds down and would only take the foremilk then fall asleep before the hindmilk came, so she needed feeding all the time.

People visited and I was still feeling like my hips were in front of me and not part of my torso. Something wasn't right and I had back pain from simply burping her on my shoulder. I felt a bit useless and not very confident trying to feed as my nipples became so cracked and sore that putting her on was agony. My boobs were not cut out for that crap and I just couldn't get her in the right position – I held her this way, did it that way, gripped the back of her neck like the nurses told me, put her on firmly when her mouth was open, got her latched on properly, fucked it up, tried again, got overwhelmed, cried, changed positions, tried a new pillow, wasted another $50 on a newly designed ring that I strapped onto my waist so Mia could feed better and didn't slip off my nipple, and I felt like Freddy Krueger had just stuck his blade into the tip of my boob! I walked around airing my nipples, oh yes, just hanging them out, no shame, no dignity, letting them heal. At one point poor Max got in the way and my nipple hit his glasses and left milk on him. I don't know who wanted to die more: him or me!

I'd had enough. I hadn't slept in days, Mia was so unsettled. It'd been three weeks. Why didn't I just get the formula?! I was so determined to master this natural ability us women have. My boobs were gigantic balloons of flowing milk and Bruno was about to go on his annual fishing trip with his best friend Dean. It was the Queen's Birthday long weekend – 8 June – and Mia was three weeks old. Remember, I'm a qualified nanny/childcare worker who already has a child and so I could handle five days on my own! I could get through it.

Bruno was a devoted father to Mia and he could pick up on her needs instinctively.

He felt guilty for going but I couldn't deny him his yearly trip away as he lights up like a teenage boy at that time of year and is the hardest worker I know. I wanted him to go and catch lots of fish. He'd held his family up and showed me such support through my pregnancy.

As I watched him drive off at 5am I felt guilty that he didn't get the perfect slim wife who popped out perfect babies and looked shagable three weeks postpartum. I saw myself as a 90kg elephant and my negative self-talk really abused me from that moment on.

Bruno was gone and Max said he felt sick. I was thinking that after seven years as an only child and only three weeks as a brother he might just need some attention. Mia swallowed up every second of my time, bless her heart, but Max felt really sick in the tummy. It was dark outside and I was feeding Mia when all of a sudden after telling my poor boy that I thought it was nothing and that he was probably just feeling new emotions about Mia arriving, he vomited all over the couch, the wooden floor, the footrest and it also hit his blanket and the side of the glass TV cabinet.

"Oh dear, I'm so sorry, Max," I said as I put Mia down and attended to my sick boy. I was frazzled. It was ridiculous really as I should've just cleaned it up and cuddled them both until they slept. Max said, "See, Mum, I told you I felt sick but you didn't believe me."

It was 11pm, Bruno was gone and the whole house blacked out. Mia was screaming uncontrollably and refused to be swaddled or lay on her back, which had been going on for days. I had pure moments of madness trying to help her. I rang Bruno and I had to go outside to the switch box in pitch black to flick the switch. No torch anywhere. No key to the flyscreen. I couldn't get out of the garage because the remote doors don't work without power. I was crying, Mia was crying and Max was asleep. I finally found a key and got it sorted but oh then the alarm had gone into saver mode and the house alarm started screeching over and over. Where's the pin to turn it off? Wouldn't work. I called security on my mobile while the alarm screamed and Mia was screaming and my brain exploded!

Once it was all fixed I begged my mother to come over. It was 2am, my mastitis erupted and I needed medicine as I had a fever, chills and felt like passing out. When my mum arrived I drove to the ER where I was given antibiotics and told to rest with a list of things to do to ease my boobs.

I got home at 5am and Mia was starving so I fed her again. I felt really strange like I didn't have a grip on myself. Moaning again, I know, but I was trying to be positive and remain a fighter.

Skip to Monday and I have Mia on formula. She sleeps peacefully but not for long and screams blood curdling sounds repeatedly! I remember gritting my teeth so hard from frustration my lip bled. It seemed to me like she was in one room and I just didn't ever have the key to open the door. She would scream on her back after a feed so I went against the rules and put her on her side on a barrier cushion so she wouldn't roll onto her face. And that helped her. She seemed to be in so much pain after feeding and I thought maybe it was reflux like Max had when he was born. I was convinced it was like a fire bubbling up her throat. Silent reflux, pure evil for babies to suffer!

Mia wouldn't settle in her bassinet. Hours of rocking that wicker hood and frame was frustrating me. I couldn't figure out why she wouldn't sleep and I always ended up putting her on my chest as the upright position was the key to her comfort. But she didn't sleep well. Daddy seemed to have noticed this too and upon coming back from his trip he also noticed she wouldn't put her neck to one side and her eyes were still sticky from birth.

We visited a cranial osteopath from a friend's suggestion that it was a lifesaver, so we gave it a go. She noted that Mia's bones in her head needed slight adjustment to help unblock the tear ducts. Just tiny bones behind her neck needed gentle holding and her eyes were never blocked again after that! You don't stop to think of that, of course. Their heads just came through the birth canal and then their skulls open after birth only to leave the fontanelle partially open.

After taking a summary of her birth, the cranial osteopath noted that due to Mia having been born so quickly her neck was out and her tummy full of wind so she was in need of a few treatments to help balance her. We noticed instant relief in Mia and she slept immediately after treatment. She is a godsend, this woman. (I wanted to kiss her and hug her but I refrained as she was too serious a woman. I usually hug everyone I meet and almost annoy them with my outward openness and affection.) Mia responded to this amazing treatment and we didn't question it.

# Chapter 9
## Light and Dark

Within two weeks of the cranial treatment I decided to take Mia to Maria for a Reiki healing session. Physically this didn't really help Mia but it did, however, help me understand her more in a spiritual sense. Her pain was raw and upsetting to see and I knew I had to try everything to help her, mind, body and spirit.

It was a sunny morning and I was happy to see my lovely caring Maria. She had sparkly eyes and was surrounded by light and love. We sat in her garden with Mia asleep in her pram as the warm breeze seemed to comfort her. I'd noticed being outside seemed to calm her mood, even if it was under the moon at 2am with the night air on her cheeks, she was calmer.

Maria and I hadn't seen each other since I was three months pregnant and Maria only knew when Mia was born through a text.

Maria placed her hands near Mia's feet and tuned into her energy. The first thing she said was, "I'm getting a strong monk vibe." She then went on to tell me that Mia is a solitary soul who chose three very emotional and sensitive people in the same family to learn affection from and to learn that it's okay to be close to people. I was a little blown away as Mia never really found comfort in my arms and generally felt uneasy. My spiritual side was lapping this up but I also had my open mind switched on too. Maria told me to sit Mia in the grass and have her near as much nature as possible because the breeze, the water and the trees are what her energy needs. But it got more interesting as Maria then said she was feeling as if Mia didn't want to be restricted: "let me out, don't swaddle me" was the message Mia was sending. Well, shit, that's what we said every day with Mia's arms outstretched above her body being what she liked. And the fact that Mia hummed all day had Maria's comment of her having monk energy really resonating with me. Maria told me Mia will teach Max strength and that her soul needs me to teach her about being affectionate and wanted as she has lived a monk life of a pure solitary existence. Call it a load of crap, but I just love the idea of looking at life through a universal energy and believing that perhaps Maria is a more highly evolved being who can teach us about our inner selves, our souls and our reason for life and heal us.

Not long after the Reiki healing session I took Mia back to our GP and was prescribed Zantac for acid reflux and to help with her constant screaming and refusal to sleep.

We were falling into what felt like a dark tunnel with our bodies having clicked into survival mode and I couldn't remember the last time I felt relaxed. I was just trying to get through it. Mia got two teeth at two months old and continued to teethe continually until all twenty teeth were out at twenty months – even her two-year molars arrived at nineteen months.

Mia had eight ear infections in fourteen months and seven lots of tonsillitis. She vomited every day and refused to sleep. She was in pain and I was helpless and fought every step of the way for her to feel comfortable. Mia was not happy and didn't find any comfort in our arms. She was only happy in a battery operated chair that vibrated and moved forwards and backwards in front of the TV. She watched TV at four months old with such commitment you would think she was an adult glued to *The Notebook* for the first time! I had noticed a certain show called *Carrie and David's Popshop*, so I taped it and she watched it all day every day and it gave me a break to breathe a little. As wrong as it was at four, five and six months old to let her watch TV, I needed a break because if she wasn't in an upright position, she was in pain, so her chair and her visual stimulation was a godsend.

My brain was going into overload as I tried to decide what to do with all my family and friends' advice on getting her to sleep. Some formed a very firm opinion that because she was now six months old and taking two hours to get to sleep it must be behavioural and she needed tough love. My heart, my soul and every part of my being told me otherwise but I tried controlled crying as well as all sorts of other things. But only Bruno and I knew what we were going through. Only a small handful of people in our lives were genuinely on our side and had seen Mia a lot and were of the opinion that she was definitely uncomfortable and that there was something going on that we just couldn't put our finger on.

Mia at seven months was about to go to sleep school as I couldn't handle another sleepless night. She was awake nineteen hours out of twenty-four. I watched this dear little girl go to bed at 7-8pm only to wake religiously half an hour later night after night screaming and vomiting until 11pm and then held upright until 12:30am or driven in the car upright in her seat until she fell asleep. We carried her in our arms and she would sleep with us, leaning over our bodies in an exhausted heap. Sleep school, I thought, that will solve all our issues, I can get the support I need and Mia can learn to self-settle in the four nights we are there with the help of trained nurses!

I arrived there and felt like we were in a very awkward place with dorm rooms for the mothers with wooden wardrobes to place our clothes in, along with a safe and key for our medicines where I had to place my antidepressants. I felt like a loony again! There were rooms for us mothers and each baby had a room no bigger than a standard bathroom with white walls, a white cot with white sheets and white curtains. Nothing colourful, nothing soothing, just a little prison for my baby to learn her new routine.

I was going to war with my child, we were going to become enemies and with trained support I would place her in her cot, walk out and leave her until instructed to go back in. Lucky for us we missed the first night as someone cancelled and so we were called in for the second day, so three nights in total.

Round one with Mia was pure hell as she screamed and vomited for the entire sleep-assisted routines. (She was in horrific stress the first night and this was no different than the final round when they decided it wasn't working for her and we should introduce each step one at a time once we got home.) After the first round I took Mia into my arms and walked outside. The blotches on her face from the stress of being left alone were resembling what I can only describe as a rash from an allergic reaction. Her lips were quivering and she looked at me with such relief to be back with my touch, my smell and my voice. I had to say bedtime and leave the room shutting the door, only returning when I noticed the cry drop into a calmer sound. If Mia was quiet when I went in I could offer a quick cuddle. If she got louder I was to walk away again, shut the door and give no eye contact.

Mia's cry never really broke or mellowed. She vomited and the nurses and I cleaned her up and cleaned the cot and they said no eye contact, no comfort, no nothing. "Get her changed ASAP and back to bed and shut the door." My body and Mia's were in terrible shock and the anxiety was unbearable! I still knew in the deepest part of my heart this was NOT behavioural for her. It was pain pain pain of some sort. But I started to question that maybe they were right and maybe I was wrong. I tried to convince myself she was just needing to be sorted. But after three nights she saw her daddy and the look on her face screamed: "get me out of here, get me out of here, Daddy, please take me home!" And so we drove so far away, so far away from getting an answer we so desperately needed.

Out of all the days with Mia these are the ones I regret so much. I would never have gone if I had known she would never break, she would never falter, she would continue to scream blue murder repeatedly over and over while left in her cot, she would vomit and vomit and vomit and after the nurses cleaned it up and taught me no eye contact was the key to her learning that she must self-settle.

To then have them decide enough is enough and that she needed me to hold her as it was not working.

She would crash in my arms upright, sobbing as if fire was burning her throat and her face was blotchy from the crying. She would sleep and again I found myself holding my girl upright, but she was getting heavier as each month passed and her constant distractions were causing her to become a very overtired baby.

We came home from sleep school with a new fear of separation that had made her worse. We vowed to never ever leave her alone again and to keep trying to get the help we so desperately needed.

*I want to be your soft place to fall. It's painful, is it, when I touch you, baby girl? Does it feel like you're always on high alert and your fidgeting and restlessness is consuming your every second? Do you feel irritated by fabrics and the slightest touch can set your skin on fire? I know you're not comfortable and I see your sheer agony when you wake and you're so rigid I can't hold you close to take it all away for you. I know your teeth hurt, your throat is sore and I'm trying desperately to get some answers for you. You don't seem to feel other forms of pain like when you bump yourself or bruise, it's like you were tickled not hurt. How can your senses do this? React so intensely to touch but not injury?*

*Mia, I will drive you to the Royal Children's Hospital at 4am. I will call the ambulance at 1:30am when you vomit and scream so much you look like you've stopped breathing. I will try and try for your answer, for only I have the power to seek it. I don't think I want to ever change you as you're my beautiful girl but I desperately want to understand you better. I'm not giving up until I find my answer.*

*I watch you repeat the same word over and over and over for it to vanish from your vocabulary only to be replaced by another single word over and over again. I hear you count beautifully from 1–20 and surprisingly in reverse and you're only fifteen months old! This is just astonishing to me how advanced you are. It's almost superhuman but a simple communication of "Mummy, drink please" or "Mia tired" you are just not saying at all. You aren't using simple comphrension in your language but you're visually a genius. Zero communication at all but an enormous amount of repetitive songs and knowledge way beyond your years. It's definitely got me puzzled.*

*I'll fight for you if it kills me. I won't stop as you're in pain and you don't deserve this, you don't have the best of me right now, I'm depleted and tired but I'm getting there and I love your skin and under your chin, I love your curls and your curious mind. I know you want my touch and you're screaming from the inside out: "Mummy, please don't go, I need you by my side, until this subsides, this pain inside and I can finally sleep."*

I felt so rejected by my baby. It was almost like she was desperate for my touch and love as I felt her want for me yet if I touched her it hurt. Even though she needed me and I could tell she did, I just knew my touch hurt her but I didn't know why yet! I kept thinking, why the hell does holding and touching her seem to really send her into overdrive emotionally? It was like my fingertips had fire on them. I felt so helpless. Mia seemed on the outside to others a naughty child, one who I knew wasn't naughty but rather strong-willed and feisty. I went over and over in my mind what this could be. Was she just stubborn and independent? I asked myself. But there was a place deep in my mind that said otherwise and as a mother I wouldn't ignore it. I would not give Mia tough love, I would not let her cry and cry and sleep in her vomit until she 'learnt'. I thought, maybe it's me who needs to learn. Maybe it's me you are teaching. I can't treat you like a textbook baby who needs behavioural therapy.

I said some dreadful things at 2am. I swore and shouted, "What is wrong with you?!" I don't think I have ever been so deeply ashamed of the words that came out of my mouth. If only we could have slept more our brains wouldn't have felt so fried. If only I could've slept next to Mia from 7:30pm until morning. I kept thinking, it's just what a child does, isn't it? Surely a child who weighs so little and is so small needs rest? If I'm feeling so tortured by lack of sleep, heaven knows how you feel.

It was also not nice to feel a big gap between Bruno and me. We hadn't slept in the same bed for months and months and months! When I was pregnant and vomiting we slept apart. When Mia was born we slept apart. When I was sick we slept apart. I missed him and he missed me. We became enemies fighting the same battle but because we only had each other to bounce off we screamed ideas at each other and we argued about what to do for Mia. We shared the task of getting her to bed at 11pm. We took turns helping each other but craved one night to just sit together alone. Our days with Mia awake were literally 7am till midnight and often until 2am, so we tried so hard to stay in check and when we did have time to make love we were transported back to being sixteen and twenty-one with fire and passion. I felt sexy and he felt my love in our moments of peace alone. It would take two or three months to get a night like that again but our love's foundation was made of solid steel and no matter what attacked it we just felt bruised and hurt but never defeated as a couple.

We were just trying to help our daughter feel at ease and content. We had made this little marshmallow, as we called her. Through our struggling to parent Mia as best we could, we had horrible fights and I hated how his vision of me was being invaded by a sleep-deprived bitch who was angry and tired and just plain awful to be around. How very sad it all was but we tried to keep our heads up as best we could. The simple things in life, like personal space were not at all taken for granted but I was also becoming so dependent on having Mia next to me to soothe me to sleep, I myself had forgotten what it was like to be independent.

One Wednesday afternoon I had been awake for days and days and days, months even, surviving on three hours a night. I remember Mia was so unsettled and I had an unimaginable frustration that if I had to rock her one more time for two hours I would go mad and I hoped I would get sick so someone would put me to bed. So I drank vodka. SO much vodka. I had my first breakdown and I broke that day into a million pieces. My mother-in-law came, my husband came home and my friend Danielle came to take me to hospital. I was in a terrible state of despair and crisis. I needed help. I scared everyone around me by laying on my kitchen floor sobbing, shouting, screaming and falling apart. I drove in the backseat of my loving friend's car and waited in the ER for two hours to see a psychologist from the wards. He listened to my situation and organised a CAT team to visit over the next two days.

It was those two days that were a godsend as the nurses who came were the first to raise an eyebrow at each other as I described Mia's symptoms and behaviours. They couldn't speculate but mentioned autism spectrum disorder. It was as if they had witnessed my world somewhere else. Like they knew exactly what I was saying. I was totally oblivious to autism. It was just a word to me, just a vision in my head of a child rocking in a corner or counting the same object over and over. This can't be Mia, I thought, she's the smartest baby I've ever met and what's this spectrum thing? I just didn't have a clue and my mind was a complete blank canvas for others to begin to paint on so I could start to understand, I'm still understanding. I knew then our relief and understanding of what was going on was not far away. But denial is a funny thing, my husband had to be on board too and this was not easy to accept. But both of us had to find out what was going on in her body and soul.

# Chapter 10
## Mia 3 Months Old

I need to rewind back to a day when Mia was twelve weeks old. It was early evening, the beginning of a new journey and one that would take a year and a half to fix. Mia was laying on the floor and I got down on the floor to kiss her and talk to her. I got up on my knees feeling sore all over still from my back. I had been to see my chiropractor who helped adjust my spine but as I went to get up I couldn't stand. Something went in my back and it was not a muscle. I didn't know what it was but if I moved my mouth it hurt. I got to my feet but was hunched over still locked this way and scared to move as it was as if my body was stuck. The pain was strange and I literally couldn't move. I said to Bruno through my teeth, "I've hurt my back, don't laugh, I'm serious." I was frightened as I just could not move.

I telephoned a few places and asked for help but I couldn't get in anywhere at 6pm and was told by nurses on call to rest in bed. From that moment on every breath I took caused a sharp pain in my spine across my midsection and into my ribs. I continued to carry on like a drama queen and visited my chiropractor the following week. He had a student in that day and he didn't do an X-ray as he said it's definitely a subluxation in the rib. He lay me on the table and adjusted where the pain was on the left side of my back right on the rib. With one sharp adjustment I felt a horrendous crack and pain. I went home in agony and felt worse!

After twelve weeks I had had enough of complaining every day. I wasn't sleeping more than three hours a night as Mia needed to be either driven or pushed in her pram to get to sleep. There was nothing I could do that would get this poor baby to sleep.

I held her night after night, in pain, rocking her in my arms in a chair and she still just couldn't get to sleep, so the car it was or a pram ride around the kitchen, lap after lap, sometimes for two hours while she squirmed and screamed and continually twisted her hair with her fingers. She was constantly distracted by the light or any distraction from me would set her back to square one. If I touched her leg or broke the rhythm there was hell to pay.

One Sunday afternoon I took myself to a bulk billing doctor's surgery and waited an hour to see a kind doctor. I told him I thought I had cracked a rib and he sent me for an X-ray. On the Tuesday I went back and he held up the X-ray and said, "You have a 6.4cm mass on your spine and a 2.7cm shadow on the lung. I'm not sure what the mass/tumour is but the shadow could be cancer. We need further tests."

Oh god. I booked into my family GP that same day and took my X-rays with me. I was sent to MIA Radiology for a CT scan and more X-rays. I was told I had a ganglioneuroma that could not be determined as benign or malignant without further tests. I was also told to see a lung specialist. Well, I shocked the hell out of my two mothers' group girls who were nurses. I think the looks on their faces as they took Mia for me so I could go to tests was priceless and masked. That worried me. I drove off thinking, well they know more than me, that's obvious, but I remained calm. Bruno was shocked and our family were too.

There's a certain numbness that clouds over you and you become your own apprentice in a mist of confusion and lack of knowledge that leaves you feeling alone.

Google and I were very close. If it wasn't Mia I was trying to diagnose, it was myself, and I actually became quite knowledgeable on certain subjects I wouldn't have learnt about otherwise.

Great things can come from bad events in our lives and I truly believe that all experiences in the world that are challenging or hard will bring a positive.

I was lucky. I was a very very lucky young woman.

Bruno and I would set off during our busy schedules to meet one of many specialists in the hope of finding out my health status. First up was the lung specialist.

I will never have the patience for waiting in stupid doctors' rooms way past appointment time. I understand that doctors are busy but holy crap can't someone chuck the *National Geographic* magazines in the bin? They should be banned. Maybe doctors' waiting rooms should have lolly jars and free wi-fi, a refreshment bar with tea or coffee facilities and some positive books on health and wellbeing. I don't care about Tom Cruise's years-old divorce from Penelope Cruz! Someone bin these magazines!

In a positive light, if Bruno wasn't there with me in these waiting rooms, I would look intently at the other patients, without them knowing, of course, but trying to guess what was wrong with them. Some were neatly dressed whilst others looked like death warmed up. Maybe they were at death's door? Don't unhealthy people float these rooms waiting to hear their fate that soon they will die from a disease or cancer? Or were they mostly going to be okay? Either way, I would guess what was wrong with them in my mind while flicking through *Woman's Day* and pretending to relax.

My first doctor lung specialist was really nice. He looked at my CT scans and decided I needed a lung biopsy at the Epworth Hospital. Serious serious stuff, Claire.

So off I went with beautiful hubby and unsettled chubby cheeks Mia to be given a pain block in the back and wait under the CT machine for another doctor to come put a long needle through my back, into my lung and into my little shadow.

I was under strict orders not to move during this procedure because if the doctor hit the wrong spot it could cause a collapsed lung. I would bleed so he would have to turn me over quickly and put another injection in my chest. So I was to stay very still so this didn't happen.

Holy crap, pardon?! I started to panic as the procedure began. I moved under the machine so he could see where he needed to navigate his needle. I never usually tremble but the fear made me tremble. I felt like crying but I just pretended I was an expert at removing my spirit self off to the beach with my toes in the sand.

"You're going to feel a bee sting now to numb your back." That was okay, but then he inserted the long wire and I felt an electric sensation in my back, moving along slowly and deeply until it reached my lung and the feeling was completely awful. It was like little robots zapping in my lung. I imagined *Transformers* (like the movie) and thought I was being invaded.

With the biopsy done and because of the radiation in the area, I was on my own to recover as no children were allowed around this ward.

While recovering I saw the tiniest old man I have ever seen on a hospital bed being wheeled in and I was shocked because it looked to me like someone had just put a mop under the blankets as all I could see was his head on the pillow. I was thrown emotionally for this man and I felt immense sadness for his suffering. I wondered what his life was like and in that sad moment I drew strength and told myself how lucky I was and that I would continue to be brave.

A chubby grumpy nurse who was dying for a coffee and to sit down told me I could leave. I was charged $1,100 for the experience.

When I received the results I couldn't even understand what it all meant. I gathered it was a clump of spindle cells and blood, but now my specialist wanted me to have a PET scan to determine if it was benign or malignant. He suggested that if it was malignant I would have to have a lower left lung lobectomy. A ... l–l–l ... what? English please? Oh, you want to cut my left lung out to save it spreading? I see, okay, well let's hope and pray it's not that then.

# Chapter 11
## Phobias

I have a severe phobia of being trapped in a confined space. The first time I came to realise this was when I was about five or six years old. I was with my family at home watching television and some old movie was on when all of a sudden the image of a man in a straitjacket came up on the screen. I had never in this lifetime seen a straitjacket yet the physical reaction I had was one of panic and I instantly remembered I had been in one! It was torture and it was frightening to have such a strong reaction to something I didn't know anything about except that I just knew I had worn one. This memory has stayed with me until this day and I've only ever seen it again in an Eminem video clip.

The next time I had a reaction to confined spaces was in Sydney at the Mardi Gras. I was walking along a street with friends and it was packed with people everywhere. We couldn't see over the metal barricades as we walked towards a street corner and from the other corner there were just as many people walking towards us. Within seconds we were trapped by people shuffling and pushing. My breathing became erratic and I could not for the life of me control it. I was unable to calm down and we fled into the 7 Eleven on the corner. While watching through the windows the pushing looked like hell and the owner of the shop was screaming for us to get out as more people were cramming in for relief. We knew we had to just get back in the crowd, hold hands and get out of the major squash of bodies and teenagers laughing and pushing people hard to make it worse. I got out with my hands above my head crying and crying, unable to breathe and in the taxi on the way home I sobbed and sobbed and said, "I'm a complete weakling."

I can't stand pain, I'm claustrophobic and I complain a lot! That night, call it my psychic intuition, I had an awful dream or possibly a memory from a past life, I'm not sure. Memories lay dormant and are triggered by an event, and with me being so empathic, I dreamt I was being transported in a van in Iraq or some desert country. I was hidden behind the number plates, which were unscrewed, and behind it under the van was a coffin-like box where people were confined. It was so horrific and so real I woke in a sweat, completely tortured by the memory that haunts me still. I've never had the guts to google this kind of act as much as I love a good google search. Me and confined spaces are a huge no no in this life with my body screaming no as my soul is reminded of it.

Off for my PET scan I'm reassured I'll be sedated, so going in the three rings will be easy and my head won't go in at all, so I'm told.

Adele was playing on the sound system to soothe me, thank god she was there with my soul, I was filled with radiation and sent on my way.

I got through it by singing in my head: *I let it fall, my heart, and as it fell you rose to claim it, it was dark and I was over, until you kissed my lips and you saved me, my hands, they're strong, but my knees were far too weak.*

My scan was about to finish as I moved further and further under in intervals and the voice overhead said two more minutes. My head went under. I was so over this suffocating feeling of not being able to control my breathing and panic, but then it was all done and I went home to wait.

Three days later I received an envelope with a copy of the CD with my results as well as my earrings that I'd left there. I thought, should I put it on the laptop and have a look for some dangerous colour on my lung that detects cancer? Oh, why not. So I googled again to make sure I knew what colour to look out for.

It was all very confusing but I concluded that I was cancer free and didn't tell anyone in my family I'd done it purely because it was a silly thing to do. We visited doctor lung specialist and he told me it was all clear and that I needed to be monitored over the next two years in case it grew. He will never know what it is and would have to cut it out to really know, but I didn't dwell on it as I had bigger problems at the minute as my spinal tumour was touching the aorta and needed to be seen by a neurosurgeon.

Mia was almost one and teething badly. She was sick on her first birthday with her sixth double ear infection and went to bed at night between 11pm and 2am. She was only sleeping six hours straight, so if she went to bed too early I could've been up from midnight till 5am with her unable to sleep. She learnt that food hurt her throat and gums with the constant teething. For seven weeks Mia ate nothing other than a little mashed banana. She was addicted to milk and had four bottles a day. We decided not to worry about it. Because she was having all that milk of course she wouldn't eat but I knew it was her one thing in life that calmed her, helped her and never hurt her. Milk for Mia was like a mother for her: a continual comfort that never let her down.

Mia's a gorgeous little girl with dark curls and a smile to melt anyone's heart. She was very clever and repeated lots of the same words over and over and over. I wasn't aware that all her behaviours were common to that of autism spectrum disorder. Not one single doctor or paediatrician ever suggested it nor did the nurses at sleep school, who with their expertise and ushering in of thousands of babies a year, you would think someone would have a clue. But no, not one person picked up on it. Mia was noted between emails as 'baffling' by one paediatrician and after waiting five months to see a gastroenterologist he said it was just a milk allergy and that she would grow out of it.

Mia was my focus. Max was fading into the background as I struggled to keep my head above water with appointments for Mia and myself. Max was no doubt affected by this awful stress and worry. In fact, he was terrified for his family as he was too young to quite understand but old enough to feel the stress of it. He needed his mummy and I did my best with him. He was so brave and helpful with Mia so I didn't need to worry too much about him. Well, not yet anyway, as his suffering would need some attention and love further down the track. I just didn't stop at the time to consider this as I had been so sleep deprived, I was unable to cope with Mia and I wish now I had been well enough to protect him more. Luckily he had lots of loving family members and two fathers to shelter him a little.

# Chapter 12
## Neurosurgeon

Another waiting room in another suburb but better magazines, and I waited to see the doctor. I recorded this consult on my iPhone as the previous few times I didn't really listen as it was all so overwhelming. Gee he was young, doctor neurosurgeon. Good looking, too. I was on my own that day and we talked about the fact that it was a slow growing tumour and that he would remove it from entering my chest but needed me to have an MRI. If I was seventy plus years of age they would just leave it, but I hopefully had fifty plus years left and the tumour was causing chronic pain when breathing so it needed to be removed.

I couldn't breathe and began to panic at the thought of slowly moving into a confined tube. I was sweating and my heart rate was going up as I told him there's no way on earth I could do that without being sedated. He was a busy man and I could tell I was being a royal pain in the arse as it would take ages to organise having to have an anaesthetist available on the same day and time. Plus I would have to pay around $800 of my own money to be put to sleep. I don't care, buddy, I'm not going in that machine awake!

So it took almost six weeks to organise and I met a few very sick people in the waiting rooms that day. One man in particular was so open about his health when speaking to me once we are ushered together for our MRI scans. He had been through the ringer and just said, "God will either need you soon or you will be needed here longer. Just pray you get to see your family grow."

Ouch, that stung as I was under the impression I was okay. I wasn't anywhere near as sick as those people. I will live to ninety plus. I will live a long life, I thought. It was just a hurdle and so I began to describe my journey from that moment on as my little life's hurdle. Nothing more, nothing less.

I was put to sleep and then woke up with a sore throat.

All done. Results! Firstly, he assured me my brain was all clear. Trying to humour me a little, hey, buddy, my brain is not okay, have you met my family? I've been kookoo my whole life. Medically it may have looked clear but it so wasn't clear. It's been pickled and scared and worried but I was glad he said it was okay. He told me he wasn't the surgeon for the job as it was touching the aorta and he would open me from the front chest wall, so he referred me to a thoracic surgeon. Keyhole was probably to be my best option. I drove home so confused and numb I got so lost I couldn't find a road that was remotely in my home's direction. I was so fed up and anxious to meet another doctor.

I drove into the city by myself and met Dr Gavin Wright, another handsome doctor with awesome magazines.

He had a gentle energy about him and even though he was a very busy man he was the first doctor that almost made me feel like a relative, as he spoke with such empathy and concern that I felt at ease. He looked at my rather large envelope of scans from my MRI that had now become my portfolio in a way – I'd always wanted a portfolio of me in the hopes of becoming a model in the future. I wanted to be on the cover of *Dolly* magazine, but this kind of portfolio contained my pictures right there in dark blue, shades of white and black peering at us on a fluorescent light.

He could see every angle of my insides, every perfect organ along with my little shadow and my hurdle. I was in his company for a whole hour! That's a lot of time for a consultation. He wanted to remove the ganglioneuroma from my spine via either keyhole surgery or by having VATS surgery at the Cancer Hospital. VATS is video assisted thoracic surgery, whereby the doctor is trained to use highly technical machinery in a capsule holding remote controlled hands while three spears were placed through my ribs. I'm sure there's a more technical description but that's my version of what I heard. I would go on a heart lung machine, meaning one lung was collapsed while the other connected to the machine.

Oh my gosh, this I did not like the sound of and I was scared a little but he needed to have space in the chest cavity to remove the tumour. He even said, shame the lung needed is the one on the machine as that's the one with my little shadow and he could have removed that while he was there, but it was on the opposite side. He looked excited by this moment in his career as I'm sure there are not a lot of surgeons doing this kind of surgery.

I instantly trusted him with my body as he was to me the Wizard of Oz and he could show me the way home to Kansas. He could take me down the yellow brick road to home. Home where Claire had been sleeping and laying dormant. He told me there was a waiting list for VATS and I chose this only as it was less invasive than keyhole. I couldn't wait to get home and google it all!

He was wearing a purple shirt with shades of blue stripes and I stared at the pen in his shirt, the look in his eyes, the way he was looking at his notes and I cried and asked if I'll be okay. He told me we won't know until it's out and whether it's malignant or even if he can remove all of it.

I was to be in hospital for five days and this to me sounded like a holiday in a resort for a week. You mean I get to lie down in a bed and rest and not hold Mia for a few days? You mean I'll be fed and looked after while I rest? You mean I'll have six more weeks of recovery? In my worn out depleted state of mind this very sad unfortunate piece of information actually made me feel excited. I realise now how sad that sounds and what state of mind I must have been in! The guilt gripped me but I pushed it to the back of me. No one wants to go to a cancer hospital, I must've been crazy to have even had that thought.

My head was cloudy, my vision strange, I saw a wiggly line like a strand of hair under a microscope in my vision, my sleep deprivation was torture as I couldn't think clearly and my words wouldn't come out. I dreamt of going to sleep and I dreamt of staying in bed all night. I wanted it like an addict wants her next hit! I couldn't believe as a mother of two children that I had these thoughts of wanting to escape, wanting to be sick and cared for. How can this hole I've fallen into be consuming me so negatively? I felt like a loony, actually someone slightly insane, and I stayed this way until I got a date for surgery: 19 April 2012. Perfect. Just after Max's eighth birthday and just before Mia's first birthday so I could be home for both.

Three days before the date my surgery was cancelled due to more needy patients. And I understood completely, but I was anxious and tired and the pain had been like a hook in my back connected to a rubber band that stretched when I was breathing. I wished to stop breathing for an hour to have a rest from the pain. It had been a year since searching for a solution and I'd had enough but I knew I could keep going for a little longer.

I didn't think I was being a happy mum around my children. My zest had all but gone as I'd forgotten to laugh and if only I could've slept so my brain could begin to repair a little. It had been eight nights in a row of poor Mia being up until after 1am. She was about to celebrate her first birthday on Sunday and her cake was very pretty: a princess pillow with her name on it. All the family were coming over and Mia was refusing to eat two days prior to the party. She never got a temperature with her constant ear infections and I could only tell as she wouldn't eat anything and touching her was impossible. I got in the car with Mia in the back seat screaming. I'd tried the pram ride for an hour in the kitchen and I'd held her as much as she would allow.

# Chapter 13
## Surgery

I had another date for surgery – June 19 2012! I was having elated feelings of joy at the thought of my body resting and I battled in my brain about how ridiculous it was but I couldn't help it. I prayed for 19 June to come.

The day arrived. It was the day I was to leave the house and begin my journey to recovery and put my life in the hands of surgeons.

I wasn't worried that three spears were to go through my ribs. What worried me more was the catheter. I find the whole concept odd. The whole idea that while I'm asleep someone is hooking my urethra up to a bag. How odd. I know it's common practice but I feel weird about it, especially after my nurse friends told me they measure it to see which size tube fits! Each girl requires a different sized tube to be inserted into her urethra. Oh the less I know the better, thanks girls! So I asked the nurse to make sure it was only a woman who put it in. Also, I was going on the heart and lung machine! That was a worry too but I didn't think about it. Much!

My in-laws were prepared to move in for the next six weeks so Bruno could work and have his mum cook. Thank god we had them to help and support us.

Bruno turned forty that week and his father turned eighty! Usually it was an important milestone in one's life and usually both those birthdays would warrant a party of some sort. I'd hoped in the future

Bruno would do something nice to celebrate his humble hardworking self and be surrounded by loved ones drinking wine and celebrating, but this unfortunately never happened for either of them. However, I hoped we could reflect on our blessings for we have life and others are a hell of a lot worse off in life than myself and my little hurdle.

The day came and the children were sorted.

I was in the preparation room putting stockings on and a really ugly gown when I thought, gee my boobs hang now without a bra! Having baby number two sure has changed things around here! I had a vision of the way they used to look and giggled to myself.

I walked along four long corridors with Bruno and then had to say goodbye. We kissed and hugged and I felt like for the first time I was looking at him and unable to read his face. I usually know all his expressions. I can tell when he is excited or nervous. I can always tell when I've pushed him to his limit and I have made him mad and I know the face he has of adoration for me, but this face as I said goodbye was one I hope not to see again. His darling sweetheart was having surgery on her spine to remove a tumour. He disappeared and was gone out of sight but I could still smell the lingering Lynx effect of his deodorant that he had left on my gown. The scent was masculine and warm and I've never been more in love with him than that moment in the ugly stale corridors of Peter Mac Hospital.

I met a lovely anaesthetist who I liked as he was calm and sincere but couldn't find a vein to save his life. Four attempts later and covered in bruises he had to call his superior in. I felt sorry for him but we finally used the left arm for the arterial line then I got a block in my back too. That was all okay and then the team arrived! Shit, a herd of what looked like *Grey's Anatomy* actors appeared all serious and they gathered around me with some talking about the surgery amongst themselves and others making me laugh to keep me calm.

I was wheeled into the VAT surgery theatre. Wowee the penthouse of theatres! This was sterile and bizarre to me. I felt like E.T. about to be examined by another interested species. I was asked what drink I would like and I said, "a gin and tonic please and with ice and a slice! Oh and could you do a quick tummy tuck if you have time?" One doctor in his scrubs laughed out loud at that comment, but I was serious.

Then I was gone.

Blackness.

Empty.

Back in five hours.

I don't remember much of intensive care other than seeing Bugs Bunny and Hugh Grant racing towards me while the walls moved and wiggled around. I heard people and saw them but I couldn't get my words out. Ketamine and god knows what else I had in my system took the pain away! I saw my mum and Bruno coming towards me but I was unable to talk to them.

The chest tube was inserted into my pleural space to collect fluid and I began to scream and scream in pain and there were five nurses around me saying it could come out whilst others saying not until I was back on the ward. I just felt very weird and had no idea what was really going on. I eventually went back to the ward and Bruno was there as they removed the chest tube easily but the pain after was quite high. I wasn't prepared for the nerves in my body to be so damaged, and the zaps, little did I know they would continue constantly for another fifteen months from my side into my left breast and striking and stopping at my belly button. It's still sensitive to this day.

I'm not going to bore the hell out of all of you as we have all at some point been in hospital and some worse off than others. Remember this was only my hurdle in life and besides the difficulty of getting through the pain, I was in a room with real life warriors who had cancer. I wasn't sure yet what my tumour was made of but I was to find out soon. I was in a room with very sick people: a mother, a grandfather, and believe it or not, a doctor was there having his bowels treated. I couldn't believe how lucky I felt as I knew deep down I'd be okay. My heart and soul knew this and I was certain of it. Friends and family visited and I was really blown away by their love and support.

It was a hard five days in hospital and even though I thought that holiday was what I wanted, that kind of 'resort-type holiday' wasn't something I truly wished for. One night in particular I had a nurse called Katie. Now she was an angel from god above. She came into my room and offered to brush my hair and put it up in a ponytail! "Yes please," I said, and the way she brushed my hair I just knew she dealt with very sick people as she made every hour of her shift important to me. As she replaced my water, filled my tissue box, wiped down my tray and bedside with lavender oil, got me a lamp, plugged it in, made my magazines neat again and in reach and even put Nivea on my face, I couldn't help but cry. Cry for the guilt I felt at not knowing yet if I had cancer and here she was spoiling me. I felt unworthy of such attention so I told her, "That's okay, you don't have to do all this, it's just me. I'm not that sick." She hugged me and said, "Claire, you have had major surgery and we have you on high doses of serious pain meds. You deserve all that I'm doing, plus, it's my job." Well, she went above and beyond for me that night and it will stay with me forever.

# Chapter 14
## Healing

Often physical healing takes place quickly compared to emotional healing. It's a different thing altogether. Scars heal, nerves regenerate, time heals all wounds. But how much time? I asked. My body healed from the scars and I began to stand on two feet again slowly. It took a year but once the heavy pain meds were out of my system and the blood pressure of my two nurse friends returned to normal from them worrying about me becoming addicted, I began to focus on my family again.

I had no time really to be allowing my husband to sacrifice work. I had no time really to sit around and mope. It was time to catch up to myself physically as that's what indicates we are healed, isn't it? Once the skin dries up and the blood is gone it's time to move on and keep going. No time for emotional wounds. They run too deep here and no amount of pain meds will ever begin to chip into the emotional pain etched so deep in me. I felt like an ocean hiding depths of pain and heartache that I left on the ocean's floor. My last few years with Mia and myself and my back were so deeply buried, I left it all thousands of feet beneath the sand and laying in the darkest ocean thousands and thousands of feet below. This emotional pain won't be sorted in front of a psychologist or a psychiatrist for $150 a session. There was no bullshit hero going to save me by talking about it all and working through it. No way could I rely on anyone else to understand my hurdle. My baby. My husband. My son. My pain. My journey. I knew it. I owned it. I felt it and I was determined to fix it, but how?

How did I get so broken so quickly with every seam on my skin torn apart? How could I make sure the good ole Clairebear awakened and bounced back to her beautiful sincere and pure self? I felt like I died that day I found out I was pregnant. I stopped that day I fell ill and vomited. I should have been able to get through it. I'm a woman and we were made to have babies, weren't we? Was it that fucking tumour that was already affixed to my spine causing the dreadful pregnancy symptoms? If I had known it was there before I might not have made myself daily feel like a failure and that I couldn't carry out this amazing gift and natural ability us woman have to be able to bear children. I had to find the lion in me. That girl who is very intuitive and knows better. I had to go to war with my soul and fight my ego driven mind of thoughts that serve me no good. My ego needed a soul cleanse. The only true way back to myself was to start thinking on a soul level with my core self and I just might come back from all this a better Clairebear, I thought. A more enlightened one closer to our great spirit himself.

# Chapter 15
## Diagnosis

Sadly I was a very angry mum. A frustrated one. Quite honestly, I was slightly resentful that my continuing efforts to comfort Mia were rejected. We were getting there slowly but Mia was still so sick with tonsils and ear infections. I was convinced that she had become numb to the pain as she just fought on. And I became numb to my life. It became a bit like a rainbow: we could only see glimpses of ourselves after it had been pouring with rain and then the sun shone.

We as a family had constant storms. I mean constant thunderstorms with sleep and illness and sensory defensiveness. It was like clockwork but only after the storm did we see a rainbow. Just a glimpse, really, enough to quickly say sorry to each other, have a cuddle and regroup for the next storm. Our lives were a constant storm and I couldn't predict if the next night I might cause the lights to go out forever. I was petrified of my own anger and my husband's in our moments of pure madness and frustration. But we would see a rainbow again. My heart bled after our storms and I couldn't figure out how to fix Mia's comforts. I couldn't help her eat better, sleep better, feel better. I couldn't calm her down, I couldn't take her out in public without her flipping her lid and freaking out, I couldn't get the house in order or run a simple life. I just couldn't figure out this simple quest and it killed me. I thought, shouldn't it be easy, even simple to live a balanced and happy life? We have the ingredients: love, commitment, honour. Why is it so hard to stop the storms from coming in our children's and family's life?

Still our Mia was awake mostly from 8am till 2am with a tiny twenty minute nap in the day. It had been nearly two years of this sleeping and screaming. Two years of utter madness. But I finally knew what I had to do; I decided to organise Mia's christening and joint second birthday. It was time to ask our church to welcome Mia into their home and hearts and celebrate being happy and healthy. We had cancelled her christening due to my operation so I wanted to get this organised and enjoy our family and friends. Living simply was a quest I continued to try to fill.

Max at this point began to feel sad every time he was due to visit his dad's for the weekend. I couldn't focus enough to figure out why. His little face fell apart into pure upset at the thought of leaving. Never in my mind did I realise it was me he didn't want to leave. I naturally thought it was something at his father's upsetting him. But he is a great father who provides a safe and nurturing home for his son. Almost like a retreat of peace for Max to go to.

One sunny afternoon we were visiting our very close friend who is into the universal energy of all things sacred and who lives a gypsy life of freedom and joy. She always said Max was in tune with his higher self. She was right as his room is filled with buddhas and gems and crystal lamps and he often feels everything like a typical empathic personality.

So this one day our friend asked Max to pray with her to Ganesh knowing he loved Ganesh and had a poster of hers in his room. He gently held his hands together in front of him and closed his eyes. He prayed out loud and these words will stay with me forever: "Ganesh, please take away my mum's worry and help Mia be happy." I knew in that instant why he didn't want to leave. I think he thought if he left he wouldn't be able to help at night in our moments of madness when getting Mia to bed. He wanted to be there for Mia to comfort her and help her too. A very deeply emotional and caring child in this family. One who wants to help and can help calm the raging storms in his mother. I had explained many times to my son about sleep deprivation and how it's very hard to stay awake for twenty hours out of twenty-four. Over and over, months and months, what a burden to have placed on a nine-year-old boy.

Max was part of this storm and he was the sun that shone on us all. Every day he was bright and warm and reminded me of why I'm a mother. I drew strength from him to give to Mia. He reminded me of my old self and allowed me to see in my mind's eye the beautiful, caring and funny mother and friend I am.

The christening was our first day of peace, love and joy as we listened to the harp player I organised and as we united with our family and friends. We ate fine food and drank wine, we laughed and cherish God's invitation of safety and love. We stood united as I read my speech and the poem I wrote for Mia. In my heart I knew and felt that the storms would pass with time and I felt inner joy that Mia was now two.

Our new home was built and our lives would only improve as we are strong and willing to never give up together. We may have lostd friends along the way through judgement but that's okay. I could deal with that. At thirty-six I was willing to let go of people who no longer served or honoured our love. The Christening was a rebirth and a death of what had been. It was time to get on with life and raise our two children as best we could, for isn't that the commitment we made when they were born? They are not trophies or toys to play with, they are individuals who need us to guide them and nurture them. I'd had enough of being angry and I wanted to find my inner light. It may take another few years of slowly trying every day but I knew I'd get there.

Mia continued to have multiple ear infections and tonsillitis infections and was plugged with more antibiotics: sixteen double ear infections and fifteen tonsillitis infections! Yet still I was focused on this mainstream idea that she had some learning delays.

Through childcare we had Mia assessed and our paediatrician was helping us figure out what was going on. He is very clever and understood her situation and could empathise with our family's sleep issues. He reassured us that no one can function like that and melatonin is still our best medicine to help Mia wind down of an evening. She was a busy two-year-old and like all her age she was emotional and fun loving.

In September 2013 our paediatrician came to the conclusion that Mia was marginally borderline on the autism spectrum disorder. I was sitting there alone with Mia next to me and a tissue that soaked the tears of shock and relief that someone cared enough to stick with us and help. His words were: "Mia is very intelligent and I'm so proud of you, Mum, as you never gave up fighting for an answer. Most parents ignore the signs and come in when their child is four or five and I say to them when did you feel this way and they say since their child was tiny!"

I wanted to explode out of the room as the last two years began flashing in my head like a horror show. I couldn't breathe. Was that what I'd been wanting to hear? Not really, but was it what I needed to hear? Yes, definitely. To hear that I wasn't going insane. That I knew she wasn't right and she was in one room and I was in the other and no matter what key I tried to unlock her door it just wouldn't open! He went on to say: "A child's brain is pliable and with occupational therapy and speech therapy these symptoms will drop off and by the time she's at school it will be as if nothing's wrong. The splinter behaviours will correct and we can help Mia. Think of it as a learning delay, if you like."

I walked the hallway to my car and placed Mia in the back seat. We left The Royal Children's Hospital and made our way home. Left then right then left … I turned wherever the car took me as I dialled Bruno's number and felt like a microwave popcorn bag exploding and steaming, but I was covered in sugar too! Sweet sugar of happiness for I had my answer. I had a diagnosis and I didn't care what anyone thought as for the first time since she was born I felt like I wouldn't ever be alone again to go through the struggles. I wouldn't ever question what's wrong and there was a whole world of knowledge waiting for me to learn. This was not an easy day. The diagnosis day. But it was the first day of the rest of our lives with autism spectrum disorder and I could be proud! I didn't think I'd ever be on the fundraising team or wearing the t-shirt as half of me clung to his words: "By the time she goes to school these splinter behaviours would have all but dropped off."

So there I was pacing my house all afternoon, bursting into tears then smiling in relief that we would be granted some funds to help our darling girl get the best therapy and I could start reading stories of other mothers like me! Shit, I didn't know there were other vampires like me! Women who never sleep and who are made of steel and can live in this world of parenting the new breeds sent to wake us up from our ignorance. Not all kids are the same. That our parents parents were wrong. That we are not all mainstream. I'm going to talk about that later but for now it was me and a glass of well-earned red!

# Chapter 16
## Compassion

Nobody wants a diagnosis of any type, do they? No one wants to be suffering or different from the person next to them. But without asking for it we were forced to except our fate and it's not until we got there we realised there's a whole world of the same type of people going through the exact same thing, just different levels of it.

It's actually better being there than being on the borderline wondering where you belong as you can start to accept things and move forward once you stop worrying about what others think.

I remember typing a letter to over fifty close friends on Facebook after Mia was diagnosed and I wasn't once ashamed of what people might've thought as I told them about Mia. I thanked them for supporting us because out of the one hundred odd people that knew, only a small handful asked offensive questions out of fear and lack of knowledge, but the rest of our friends and family offered sincere words of love and support. It was like a blanket of colourful well wishes washed over me and their words of encouragement about who I was as a mother and friend gave me so much strength and pride and helped keep me marching on.

I was advised to just call it a learning delay and that Mia would catch up by age five or six but I knew the splinter behaviours were enough for now to claim this diagnosis. Given her extremely independent and highly sociable skills it was very contradictory to the typical list of ASD symptoms. But there were three major issues here, which were undeniable sleep sensory, advanced intellect and Mia always being unwell. We also had the added faith that once her tonsils and adenoids were removed and grommets put in she would thrive. But it was only 2013 and she was just beginning her therapy and too young for such an operation, or at least we hadn't been advised to do so ... yet. However, it was an invitation to sanity land awaiting us and a chance for our family's storms to calm right down long enough for sun to shine continually and warm our hearts and bring peace to our loving family. Mia deserves health. Max deserves health. We all deserve true wellbeing.

What others think should never sway you in life. I know it does. It always does especially more so by those we love. It's often our dearly loved parents whose opinions of us mean the most. I haven't mentioned my own parents a lot as that's enough for a second book, but I will say that I know they love me very much and I know they are proud of me and I also know I have far exceeded their expectations as far as motherhood goes and I know they are in awe of my strength and compassion for my family. But their opinions of me have been the most important often without me realising until later, but every single word they say to me (yes even though I'm thirty-six) goes into my soul and embeds itself into the core of my being. It has held such weight and often put me under too much pressure to be more. More than I already am. And what I mean by that is their judgement of me has caused me so much anxiety. I felt like I was failing because Mia wasn't what she ought to have been. Mia wasn't what we all expect a baby to be. Mia wasn't calm and abiding. Mia wasn't well-behaved. Mia wasn't a good sleeper. But she was mine and I had to do what I felt was right for me and that was to stick to my inner voice telling me something was wrong and that it wasn't just naughtiness, which was hard.

I didn't want to look fat and unhealthy in my parents' eyes. I didn't want to fall behind and lose my coping skills. I didn't want to be sick and go to hospital and have to ask them for help. I didn't want to have to explain to them about autism. I didn't want to explain my struggles.

I didn't want to say I needed them because truth be told they needed me too. I was a pillar of strength for them too as I was the one they needed for advice and I felt like I let them down.

So Mia's diagnosis and my diagnosis brought me to a place of freedom and great healing as it stopped me parenting my parents and it stopped me worrying about mainstream old-fashioned parenting beliefs that are embedded in our parents from the generations before them. I stopped holding everyone up and started holding myself up and my children. I had to let go of trying to please everyone by putting myself under enormous strain in public with them. I could feel the stress and anxiety build when arriving with Mia at any family event, hoping that she would be the perfect calm child and I would handle it calmly. I learnt that part of being on the spectrum was not coping with change and public outings being extremely overwhelming, which was the case for Mia, and that a meltdown was totally different from a tantrum. It is a very hard experience to get through as when a meltdown takes place you only wish to god no one ever ever sees it, especially family. I learnt so much through Mia's diagnosis about the body and the mind and sensory defensiveness that I was becoming more compassionate towards Mia and her daily struggles. My parents are very proud of me for sticking to my beliefs and I know they love us very much.

So no, we don't want to be diagnosed in any way and we don't want to be judged and all we crave at any age is compassion. We want to be equal and understood. We want health and peace and people and family in our lives that shine understanding our way and hold us up when we fall. It's not always possible but it's what we all want, otherwise we wouldn't fight for it so much.

# Chapter 17
## Wisdom

I'd all but closed off from my connection to spirit and all that universal energy I so desperately needed. I couldn't sit still, I couldn't relax and I couldn't meditate to save my life. Deep inside my soul craved it but I couldn't find time to connect. How beneficial it would have been to meditate for just a few minutes a day but I was still a bag of crazy and couldn't stop long enough to begin to relax from feeling depressed, moody and angry and frustrated as every week was like crazy town and I kept missing the train ride to peacefulness and stillness.

I wasn't giving up, however, as my yearning to do Reiki or become a practising medium was still so strong in my heart and I knew that through all this I could become ready for the next stage of me. Not mother, not wife, not friend but the next stage of ME. Who I am. Who I am in my core. And that's what I wanted to find to become the best me. If I stayed stuck in anger and depression I'd be trapped forever and my kids didn't have the best of me at that time but I refused to die in that moment in my life as I was determined to survive it and become the most calm reflective and wise woman I knew I could be.

What makes us wise? Is it getting through each experience in life then rethinking what we learnt from it and actually putting it into action? Words are cheap but actually behaving and changing on an emotional level really takes a conscious effort.

My marriage was depleted and hacked into by ourselves. We took for granted the glue that bound us. When I looked at Bruno in the struggle with our child I forgot to notice the young man I fell in love with and it wasn't that I didn't want to, it was just that I couldn't see a clear day. I couldn't find a moment in my life anymore to think of him that way and he couldn't see me that way either. Two people ripped into shreds and hanging on. What kept us from slipping forever is the love between our souls. The deep connection that was formed twenty-odd years ago that sucks us into a time machine when we make love. Not a second is lost under his embrace and his touch reminds me I'm safe and faith is restored. I'm simply not prepared to lose it and I make a conscious effort to be kind.

You may all be thinking, what the fuck is she going on about? How can having a child ruin a marriage? How can raising kids be such a burden? But I'm here to write my reality of how hard it was for me to raise a child I assumed would fit into society's classic box of normal and how shocked we were when she was everything but classic. She was unique and strong and a warrior who was dealing with illness and sickness. I thought that parents were the strong ones teaching our young how to survive and protecting them but Mia took us for a ride into her existence of pain. Earaches, reflux, sensory defensiveness and sleep issues and there's nothing more painful for a parent who can't help their child. No matter how hard it was to keep asking and going to different doctors knowing something was amiss but hitting a brick wall every time. Holding her night after night while she suffered, I'm so grateful she is now three and a half and that this story ends well.

Our storm does finish when Mia turns three years old and two months.

I get my future diagnosis and we are all born again. This is the beginning of the end of my book.

# Chapter 18
## Moving Forward

Our Peadiatrician took a sincere genuine interest in Mia not because it was his job but because he does his job with his heart. He took charge and decided Mia needed to see an ENT specialist and that she had suffered enough. His words were: "Let's get those tonsils out. You could just reach in and pull them out they are just so big."

Mia's ears were tested and her hearing was below average and there was fluid trapped behind. No wonder she couldn't hear or develop normally. No wonder after seventeen bouts of double ear infections she would be showing autistic traits. No wonder after sixteen bouts of tonsillitis she would be sick from eighteen priscriptions of antibiotics some of which were pure penicilian.

So as I said I'm a simple woman and some might say otherwise. Some might say I'm borderline crazy or that I can't write too well. But I don't mind how you see me for that's your truth and that's beautiful and real for you. I'm just a girl who grew into her remarkable life with an ever evolving growth of her soul and I think that's all we can hope for. And that our children are happy and healthy and our lives are fulfilled.

As I finish my book tonight I'm now thirty-nine and Mia is five and a half years old and ready for school. She has overcome so many obstacles. She is even classed as being unable to be put on the spectrum due to her progression and how she is exceeding her abilities on so many academic levels. She is, however, and will always display splinter behaviours and sensory defensiveness. Whether she's on that spectrum or not we are all in it together and Mia is nothing short of confident with a thirst for life. Nothing holds her back socially and she's fiery and independent. What more could I want? After her operations she hasn't had any more infections in her nose, ears and throat and therefore was able to slowly, in her own time, catch up with her peers!

# Chapter 19
## Conclusion

Oh, I'm back again! Mia's now about to start Grade 1. It's 2018 and her prep year was mighty incredible as she soared through her work and was truly part of the furniture, so to speak! Mia loves school, has sensory overload, often rips all her clothes off after school in the car and we sail home whilst she's in her undies in the backseat free from clothes with the wind in her hair like the little free spirit she is.

Mia and Max are incredible humans who came through me. My job is to raise them, respect them and never quit on them. We all fight this fight and wouldn't have it any other way. I'm no different from the next mother as we are all fighters. We are fierce and always always get through the storms and what beautiful weather awaits each time that storm is over!

I send you all my love.

You got this.

Now I'm off for a nanna nap.

Don't wake me up xxxxx

# About the Author

Claire Gissara is a qualified practising Reiki healer and spiritual medium. Born in the East End of London in 1977, Claire now lives in Victoria Australia with her husband Bruno and two children Max and Mia. A compassionate caring woman with a love and passion for meditation, Reiki, mindfulness and mental health care, Claire has always had a desire to help others and remind people that we are all on the path to awakening and finding inner peace.

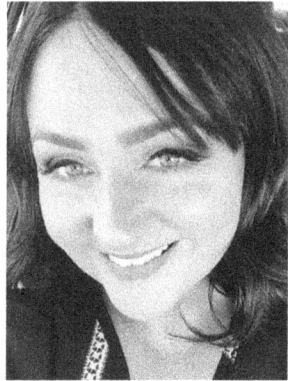

www.ingramcontent.com/pod-product-compliance
Lightning Source LLC
Chambersburg PA
CBHW020008290326
41935CB00007B/348